Under the Stars

Romances for Seniors

∽

seniorality

Under the Stars -
Jamie Stonebridge, Tiffany Martin

Copyright © 2024
Seniorality / Everbreeze Media Oy

This is a work of fiction. Names and characters are the product of the author's imagination and any resemblance to actual persons, living or dead, is entirely coincidental.

Set in 23 pt EB Garamond

Chapter 1
The Adventure Begins

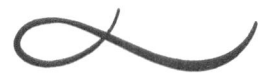

THE SMALL TOWN of Newhill had always been a place Milly found relaxing.

Her job as a receptionist in town for the local accountant paid the bills, but it was not what she really wanted in life. Besides one day having a family, she hoped to visit as many beautiful places as possible.

She felt like she would settle for visiting places as her dream of having a family didn't seem possible for her right at that time.

"Are you excited for your hiking trip this weekend?" Darlene, Milly's coworker, asked.

"Beyond excited! I have everything packed - well, almost. I just need to put a few more things in my backpack that I picked up from the grocery store. I found this awesome new granola bar to try out," Milly explained excitedly.

Darlene gave Milly a confused look. Excitement over a granola bar? Milly certainly thought so. She shrugged as she flipped the latest folder over and put it away tidily.

"It's a good thing you're pretty," she smiled at Milly and turned back to her work.

There was only one more hour to go before Milly could set off for her trip. She had been told that the Kisik Grotto was one of the most beautiful places within a short drive from where Milly lived. However, many might find a two-hour car drive to be too long, but not Milly.

Milly had always enjoyed being outside and exploring her beautiful country's diverse landscape.

Where she lived, the lands were covered in trees of all kinds. During the fall, the trees turn colors spanning the spectrum of oranges, yellows, gold and red. It was magical to walk around town in the fall and watch the leaves wave in the breeze.

There was nothing like nature. It was peaceful and quiet but also filled with excitement as animals scurry about their daily lives.

It was the beginning of June, and though it was a bit cooler than you would expect for the time of year, it was the perfect time to go camping. The mosquitos weren't out and about quite yet, which was good because Milly hated getting bitten by mosquitoes.

Lunchtime finally rolled around, so Milly could head home to start her trip.

"Please be safe! I know you are a very capable twenty-five-year-old woman, but it still scares me you going up there all by yourself," Darlene said.

Darlene was a wonderful, caring woman who was nearly sixty and hadn't left town very often. She cared for Milly like she was her own daughter and understandably feels concerned for her well-being.

"I will, Darlene, I promise. I have already given my route to my parents, and I have this awesome Garmin GPS that tells me where I am, updates my parents, and in case of an emergency, I can hit a single button, and someone will come get me," Milly had explained.

She hoped the extra-long explanation would give Darlene peace of mind.

Though she knew she didn't have to, Milly appreciated how much the people around her cared.

Darlene seemed satisfied with the answer and hugged her tight before she left. Milly was happy to head home and grab her things.

Backpack - check. Hammock - check. Sleeping bag - check. Water bottle - check. Milly checked off the items on her list and added each one to her backpack.

"Don't forget the granola bars," she muttered to herself as she ran to the kitchen to grab them. After she had checked her list another five times, she put her things into her car and hit the road.

Newhill may be beautiful in its own right, but Milly loved the beauty of the parks in the area. Kisik Grotto was visited by thousands of people every year to see the gorgeous rock formations and enjoy the crystal clear water.

Milly had never been to this particular spot before and she was excited to explore the area.

Hiking alone wasn't all that frightening for her; she had been camping regularly since she was little. She and her father often took camping trips together to enjoy the great outdoors. Her favorite part was lying on her back and looking at the stars.

Being so far away from the pollution of city lights - even town lights- the sky was a sea of little stars shining down on the people of the world.

Pulling into the parking lot, Milly parked and climbed out of the car. Taking a deep breath, she breathed in the fresh air the trees provided. The gravel crunched under her hiking boots as she opened the back door to grab her bag.

She set off for the trailhead with her backpack strapped securely over her shoulders and around her waist. Milly passed a few others in the parking lot but hoped the trail would be quiet instead of busy.

The sun had already started to go down in the sky, but the hike from the parking lot to the camping platform wasn't all that far.

Milly thought she should get to it within an hour, with just enough time to set up camp. Her boots crunched the dry leaves and snapped stray branches as she followed the trail. Birds were singing and fluttering through the trees as she took in the beauty and quietness of the woods.

Milly had always loved hiking but had also wanted to find a hiking partner. She wasn't exactly introverted but also not extroverted. She enjoyed spending time with other people, but unfortunately, not many of her friends found hiking a twelve-mile trail an exciting prospect.

At one point, Milly hoped to find a partner to do these things with, but the men in her town were more into sitting in the woods hunting rather than hiking the trails.

Her mom often said that she would meet the right man at the right time one day, but Milly wondered when that would be. She was only twenty-five, but she deeply desired to settle down and spend her life with someone.

The hike was quick, barely even a hike, more like a walk, Milly thought to herself, as she made it to her camping platform.

This backcountry site wasn't the only one, as there were three other platforms pretty close by. Seeing as the area had bears, there was a shared food storage tree with a rope to lift campers' food high off the ground.

Milly had always been a hammock girl. She saw a survival show once when she was younger and figured she would try it out. She knew tenting was fun, but once she tried hammocking, she had never looked back. Just one night, spent swinging between trees had convinced her there was no better way to sleep in the woods than swinging between the trees.

The national park had a 'no campfire' rule for backcountry camping, so she used her small camp stove to heat up a tin of water to make her instant noodles and eggs.

Eggs on the trail might sound a bit excessive, but Milly loved a good egg, and after finding an egg carrier designed for camping, she didn't have to agonize over whether to bring them or not.

Milly sat beside her little stove, stirring the noodles as they cooked and looked out over the view before her. The spot she had picked was certainly beautiful.

You could see the massive lake over the tops of the trees. The campsite sat on the side of the hill and gave her the perfect view of the woods below and the lake sitting behind that.

The sun was starting to set now, and the light from the sun danced on the surface of the water; gorgeous yellows, oranges, and purple streaks floated across the waves. The wind had picked up a bit, but it was not cold.

"Amazing," Milly said into the wide-open space as she admired the beauty of the place. This was the perfect end to the day, she thought.

Milly took the noodles off the stove and replaced them with her stainless steel cup to make a cup of tea. With the sun nearly gone, Milly looked forward to her first night under the stars.

Chapter 2
Getting Out of the City

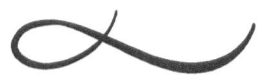

"ARE YOU SURE, Ben? You can't come?" Jay held his cell phone up to his ear as he looked over his stuff again.

"Unfortunately, Sarah isn't feeling well, so I need to stay home and be with the baby. She said she would be fine, but I can tell she isn't doing well," Ben explained.

He was a good guy, a data analyst like Jay. They had become firm friends when they figured out – over a coffee break – that they both enjoyed camping.

They had taken a few shorter trips, but this was supposed to be a big one, where they hiked to a campsite and did a longer hike the following day.

Both Jay and Ben had spent time training to make the twelve-mile hike, but unfortunately, it looked like Jay was going to be going on his own.

"I get it. You take care of that cute baby and Sarah. We'll plan another trip later in the year. I'll see you Monday." Jay finished pulling the drawstring on his backpack and moved the phone over to his other ear.

"Sounds good. Take lots of pictures. I've heard the grotto is amazing," Ben said, unable to suppress a smile as he thought about seeing it. Jay had also read that there was a hidden cave pocket in the second cave opening. He was hoping to explore it.

"Maybe next time," said Ben as Jay hung up the phone and grabbed his backpack.

Stepping out of his apartment building, he made his way over to the overpriced parking space beside the building.

City life was a means to an end for Jay. After attending college for a diploma he didn't use, he had accrued a mountain of student debt, so getting a job was a priority. He got an entry-level job in a big corporation in the city at the tender age of twenty-two.

Fast forward six years, and he was still living in the same cramped apartment, but he was climbing the corporate ladder; he was now a senior data analyst. It was well paid, but not as exciting as it sounds.

Jay went to his car, tossed his pack into the back, and climbed into the front. Only a two-hour drive separated him from a weekend of peace.

He no longer had to listen to the cars driving by and honking at all hours of the night, but instead was looking forward to hearing the crickets singing their song for their mate.

Breathing out, Jay put the car in drive and headed for the Kisik Grotto.

As Jay pulled into the park's parking lot, soft rock music played through the car stereo. Already, the tension of the city was starting to seep out of his body. With an excited push of the door, Jay was out of his car and loaded up with his backpack, making his way to the trailhead.

Jay passed a couple coming out of the trail just as he headed in.

"Just starting your hike?" the middle-aged man asked.

"Yup! Heading to the grotto tomorrow." Jay tugged on his straps a little to make sure they were secure.

"The Grotto is beautiful. We make a hike every year to see it; it's that amazing," the wife said.

Jay still couldn't believe how friendly hikers were. It surprised him when he first started hiking; living his entire life in the suburbs and then in the city, the culture wasn't overly social.

In the suburbs, you could say 'hi' to neighbors but wouldn't go out of your way to greet someone.

The city was worse; however, even a small wave received looks of confusion and an expression that said, 'Yeah, we don't do that here.'

The worn path felt good to follow and it seemed to make him think about all the possible people who could have walked the same path before him.

Jay pulled out his map to make sure he was going in the right direction. It shouldn't be all that hard for him to navigate as there were signs pointing you in the right direction, and the park gives you a map to show you where your campsite was located.

Jay and Ben had planned on a backcountry site for the first night. The spot overlooked the lake, and many of the reviews said it was a nice place to camp.

Jay enjoyed the quietness of the woods; it reminded him again of how much he wanted to get out of the city.

If Jay could pick his dream life, it would be living somewhere away from the city, in a small town, and raising his own family.

When he was growing up, he did have a stable home and good parents, but they never really did a lot together, and one thing he wanted was to have a family that had adventures with each other. Maybe one day, Jay thought.

The forest was quiet as Jay continued to follow the path. He hadn't seen anyone since the start of the trail, not that he minded.

Jay briefly saw two squirrels chase each other up a tree, the branches hitting each other as one squirrel jumped across between the trees above. Jay couldn't help but smile as he walked under the trees.

A noise to his left drew his attention. Jay caught sight of a snake on the ground. He knew it was safer to stay well away from the snake. Giving the snake a wide berth, Jay managed to avoid it without a problem.

Finally, Jay came to the top of a hill where he expected there would be a few other reserved camping pitches a way down the path. He was anxious to get set up and watch the sunset to mark his first day of hiking.

As he got closer, he could smell food in the air. Jay was not alone in this section of the park. Hopefully, he would get along with his camping neighbor.

Chapter 3
New Neighbors

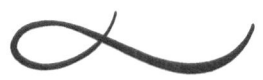

As Jay finally reached his pitch, he removed his backpack and put it on the ground. Being neighborly, he took the small path to see who else was staying in the area. Jay was momentarily speechless when he saw a beautiful woman with chocolate brown eyes.

"Hi! I'm Milly, your camping neighbor!" she said.

Her happy presence made Jay smile.

"Hey, I'm Jay. Nice to meet you."

Milly smiled at him and gave a small wave.

"You made it just in time to watch the rest of the sunset. This location is amazing," she said.

Jay turned to look out at the scene. The warm sunset cast an orange and red glow across the sky and the water.

"I'd better set up my tent quickly before I lose all the light," he said after a moment.

Milly shifted the tin of food in her hand as she adjusted to look at Jay.

"You're welcome to come and chat after you're all set. I'm boiling water for some tea, though maybe that's not exactly appealing." Jay could tell Milly was nervous about asking him that, but he also found it a little cute.

"I'd love to. Be right back." Jay hurried over to his pitch and quickly put up his one-person tent.

He had planned to eat cold leftovers for supper, so he grabbed the food container and a tin cup, which he filled with water. Maybe he could use Milly's camp stove, he thought.

By the time he was able to return, Milly was just about to sit down again.

"Hello again. I was putting my food in the storage tree over there." She pointed in the opposite direction to Jay's tent. "There are three more lines, so that you can use one as well." Her smile was shy and sweet, which Jay found very endearing.

"Thanks, I'll do that after I eat. May I join you?" Jay motioned to a rock off to the side of her little camp stove, and she nodded in agreement.

After sitting down, Jay popped open the lid of his container and stabbed the lasagna he was planning to eat for supper.

"Have you done this hike before?" Milly asked.

Jay looked up at Milly, while quickly trying to swallow his food.

"No. This is the first time I've actually done such a big hike. A friend of mine was supposed to come with me, but he had family issues to deal with. Have you hiked this before?" he asked.

Jay tried to put another piece of lasagna in his mouth, but it was getting difficult to see with the sun nearly fully set.

"Nope, this is my first time. I live about two hours away from here, so I have seen many of the smaller parks in that area, but I have wanted to see the grotto for years. I mean, the pictures alone were enticing enough to bring me all the way out here."

Milly was enjoying having someone to talk to.

"Same. I was also reading about the cave system underneath the grotto that sold it for me," Jay added.

"The cave system! I hadn't heard about that. I can't wait to get there tomorrow." Milly took a sip of her tea before turning back to Jay. "Do you know what path you are taking tomorrow?" she asked.

Jay nodded and handed her his map from his pocket. It was a bit old-school using a paper map, but Jay liked having the physical copy. "Yup," he said.

She took the map and pulled out her flashlight to see the path Jay had marked out.

"This is the same route I'm taking, too. Wanna hike it together?" she suggested.

That one comment made Jay really happy. He wasn't sure what it was about Milly that felt so right, but he liked the idea of spending all day tomorrow with her.

"Yeah, that sounds great."

Jay couldn't see Milly's face at this point due to the darkness, but he could hear the smile in her voice when she said, "Great!"

By this point, night had fallen, and Jay had finished up his supper. The stars had finally come out and lit up the sky. It was beautiful.

You couldn't see stars like this in the city. Sometimes, Jay could see some stars where he lived if it was dark enough, but most of the time, the stars hid behind the many street lamps that decorated the city.

Milly sighed from somewhere in the darkness, and at first, Jay didn't know if it's a good or bad sound, but then Milly spoke.

"I can't get enough of this sight. Looking up at the stars always reminds me how vast the universe is. We are a tiny speck in the great scheme of things, aren't we?" Her voice was wistful as she leant back and looked at the stars.

Jay thought on her words as he also looked up at the sky. She was right, and for the first time in a long time, he had finally found some peace in his busy world.

"What do you do for a living? Or are you lucky enough just to hike and explore nature?" Jay asked.

"I'm a receptionist for an accountant in my hometown. It's not an overly glamorous job, but it pays the bills, and I like who I work for, so it's pretty great all in all," said Milly.

A pang of discontentment floated around in Jay's chest. He wondered what it would be like actually to be content with where he worked, heck, just to be happy.

"What do you do?" Milly asked into the darkness.

"I'm a senior data analyst for a big corporation in the city. It's, it's not the greatest job, but it pays the bills." There was a pause before Milly spoke again.

"You don't seem very happy about that," Milly observed, her voice sounding gentle in the evening air.

Jay pushed out a breath before responding to her perceptive question.

"Like I said, it pays the bills but it's not enjoyable. I got a job quickly out of college, and I guess I never stopped to think about what I wanted. I'm twenty-eight now and have just recently realized I don't want to be in the city anymore. It's a fast-paced life that works for some, but I want something different… quieter. Maybe that's why I enjoy camping and hiking so much. I feel connected with this more than I do with the hustle and bustle of city life."

Jay felt good finally saying things out loud that he had thought for many years.

"Sounds like you need a change. Maybe this hike will help put everything into perspective for you. To see things in a new light and decide on something different," Milly suggested.

Jay couldn't help but smile at her genuine concern. She barely knew him, yet she hoped for the best for him, showing authentic kindness. Jay wasn't sure when was the last time anyone - and certainly not a woman- had genuinely cared to ask him such questions.

Something stirred in Jay, but he pushed it aside. Right now, he wanted to savor the twinkling stars above and the gentle sounds of nature around him.

"I'm glad I have met you, Milly. I think this is going to be an enjoyable trip," Jay said.

"Me too," Milly replied softly.

After a while, Jay returned slowly to his tent. With his headlamp on, he retrieved his food and walked over to the food storage tree to stow it away safely.

As he passed by Milly's pitch on his way back, he noticed that it was quiet, except for some faint movements, perhaps from her sleeping bag.

"Goodnight, Milly," Jay called out into the inky darkness.

"Goodnight, Jay," she replied softly.

A lightness settled in Jay's chest as he finally crawled into his tent.

The night time insects created a symphony of sounds, with crickets calling for their mate. It was a peaceful ambiance. Maybe Milly was right, Jay thought to himself. Maybe he could find the change he needed on this trip.

With that thought in his mind, he closed his eyes and drifted off into one of the best sleeps he had in quite a while.

Chapter 4
As Friends

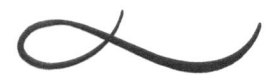

MILLY never slept in while camping, seeing as her hammock didn't block out the sunlight, but she wouldn't want it to anyway. Unzipping the net around her hammock, she tossed her legs out the side, searching for her boots.

The dew covering the ground sent a waft of freshness into the air as Milly took in the morning.

Milly started up her small camp stove and boiled some water for her oatmeal. It was full of carbs, which she knew she would need for her long hike today. Milly's stomach flipped as she thought about the day ahead. She wasn't exactly sure what she was thinking, inviting Jay to hike with her, but she was excited.

Often you find couples or groups hiking around, not typically single hikers, but it's not entirely uncommon, which was evident with Milly hiking on her own. But when she saw Jay come around the corner, she couldn't help but be surprised by how attractive he was.

He was easy to talk to, which was unusual for Milly, seeing as she wasn't exactly the most extroverted of people.

That being said, she was excited about the hike and getting to know Jay better. With the water now boiling, Milly took it off the stove and dumped a couple of packets of oatmeal into the little pot she had.

She could hear a branch breaking, drawing Milly's attention just as Jay walked around the corner.

"Good morning," Milly said as she stirred her oatmeal.

"Good morning. How did you sleep?" Jay came and sat on the same rock as he did the night before, with a small pot of his own in hand.

"Amazing!' exclaimed Milly 'I love sleeping in my hammock. I might give up my bed for a hammock permanently, if I wasn't so attached to it', she added with a smile.

Jay looked over at Milly's hammock and seemed to assess it.

"I've never slept in a hammock before. Do you prefer that over a tent?" he asked.

Milly bubbled with excitement over one of her favorite topics. "I LOVE sleeping in hammocks. The slight swinging helps me fall fast asleep. I can't believe you've never tried one. Once you have tried it, you will never go back to sleeping on the cold, hard ground."

Milly tried to tamp down her excitement as she thought about her enthusiasm for hammocks.

"You might've sold me on trying it out. I only have a small tent, which has done me well the past couple of years. Are you still happy to have me tag along on your hiking trip?" Jay asked.

"Of course! It'll be fun to have company. No one I know really enjoys this sort of thing, so it will be fun to talk to a real person instead of the animals… that sounds weird."

Jay burst out laughing as Milly fidgeted with her oatmeal pot, but her anxiety subsided when he smiled at her warmly.

"I kind of want to see the conversations you have with the animals," he joked.

The smile on Milly's face was starting to ache; she hadn't smiled this much in a long time. Not because she wasn't happy, just that she hadn't had a lot of fun times, at least in this way.

"Oh, you know, just talking about filing systems or about transcribing documents," Milly laughed. "I don't get out much, I guess."

Milly and Jay finished eating and packed up their things to set out on the long day of hiking.

It was still early enough to hear all the morning birds chirping and flying through the trees. Milly couldn't help but daydream as she walked, listening to nature.

It wasn't until they had walked for about forty-five minutes that Jay spoke up from behind her. She was walking in front because she seemed to know better where to go than Jay.

"So you said you lived in a small town. Did you camp a lot then growing up?" he asked.

"Yeah, I did. My dad took me camping all the time growing up. It was just a basic car camping experience, but it's what helped me fall in love with sleeping outdoors and hiking. Dad wasn't a huge fan of the long hikes I go on. He said he was too old to trek around in the woods like I now do."

Milly laughed. "Did you camp when you were growing up?"

"No. I grew up in suburbia. My parents weren't really outdoorsy people. We traveled a bit, but my parents worked a lot, so the idea of going away for a camping trip wasn't something that would have appealed to them. It wasn't till I met my coworker a couple of years back that I first tried it out and loved it," replied Jay.

Milly enjoyed the hike; she and Jay talked about their childhoods and what jobs they did. Milly discovered that Jay had become unsatisfied with his life in the city and had seriously been considering a change.

Milly wondered if he was afraid to take the leap, but she didn't know him well enough to make that comment.

They had hiked over three-quarters of the trail when Milly started heading down a slight hill. The path was straightforward after that, leading them to the grotto. Just before she got to the flatter part of the path, Milly's boot got caught under a loose root and she started falling forward.

Milly let out a small screech, throwing her hands out in front of herself to break her fall, but she never hit the ground. Jay had come up quickly behind her and wrapped his arm around her waist, preventing her from falling face-first onto the hard ground.

Milly's heart beat faster as she tried to catch her breath and recover from the scare of almost falling. She turned her head to look over her shoulder and was struck speechless by the hazel eyes looking down on her. Her heart skipped a beat at the tenderness she saw in his eyes.

Had Milly ever felt this before? No, she hadn't. She was struck by how comforted she felt wrapped up in Jay's arms. 'This is new,' she thought.

"Are you okay?" Jay said, a hint of concern woven into his words.

"Yes, thank you. You were quick," Milly said in a slightly shaky voice. Jay smiled at her as he helped her stand upright again.

"Wouldn't want to see someone so precious get hurt," Jay replied, his tone warm and reassuring. Milly's heart skipped again, and her cheeks reddened at the comment.

She knew she found Jay handsome but never really thought he would reciprocate an interest.

"Thanks," Milly said softly before adjusting her straps again. "Not too far now. Maybe another hour, and we should be at the grotto."

"Sounds good," Jay replied. He adjusted his pack and fell behind Milly again.

The hour-long hike went by quickly, and before they knew it, they were cresting over a small hill to see a large rock formation hanging over the clear water below.

Milly couldn't help but take a sharp breath at the sight before them. The rock formation created a half-circle, and towards the bottom of the rock, there were at least two entrances into the cave.

She stopped just at the edge as Jay came up beside her. He, too, looked at the clear blue water splashing up against the rocks.

"It's beautiful," Jay remarked. Milly quickly agreed. "Want to head down?" Jay looked over at Milly.

"Yes!" Milly jumped in excitement, despite the hours of hiking they had already done.

The path to the bottom was steep, which made Milly a little nervous, considering she had nearly fallen an hour earlier. She really didn't want a repeat performance in front of Jay or into the depths of this beautiful natural space.

Jay must have noticed her hesitation because he reached out his hand for Milly to take without much thought, so they could hike down to the bottom together.

His hand was warm and strong, which made little butterflies take off in her stomach. The feeling of something new had started, and Milly was excited to see where it would go.

At the bottom, they walked along the narrow path to the first open cave, where the water reflected colors off the cave ceiling.

It was magical, and Milly couldn't take her eyes off everything around her. A couple of times, she caught Jay watching her; he never hid it. He would just smile at her and look around as well.

"So the hidden cave is just over here. Do you want to take a look?" he asked.

"Are you kidding! Of course, I do." Taking his hand again, she followed him a bit further into the second cave, walking around a corner that didn't look like a corner. It appeared more like a wall, and if you didn't know it was there, you would have missed it.

A small stream followed their path, and the hidden cave appeared within a minute.

Milly gasped at the sight. A hole in the top allowed a shaft of daylight to pour in from above, casting a bright spotlight on the crystal blue water.

"Want to sit for a while?" Jay asked.

"Sure," she replied.

Quickly, Milly removed her pack and set it down against one of the walls. There was a ledge big enough to sit on and put your feet in the water.

Milly wasted no time removing her boots and rolling up her pants to dip her feet in the cold water.

Jay did the same. Milly figured he would sit a bit away from her, even though she wanted to feel his gentle touch again. To her surprise, he came and sat right beside her, his leg gently touching hers as they sat.

The moment was beautiful, and Milly would remember it always. The two of them, the beauty of the hidden cave, and being in that moment was wonderful.

Before too long, they put their shoes back on, grabbed their packs, and headed out of the grotto towards their next camp site.

The connection between Milly and Jay was real, and Milly wondered if this was just a magical weekend or if it would be more than that one day.

Chapter 5
Under the Stars

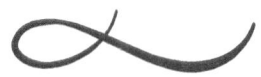

JAY had reserved another camping pitch, but it was situated farther away from Milly's site. However, he felt a strong desire to remain close to her.

When he mentioned this to Milly, she generously offered him to join her in her area which was much larger and could accommodate up to four people.

Jay might have shown a bit too much enthusiasm in accepting her offer, but

Milly's beaming smile assured him that she was pleased he agreed.

Milly's pitch had a fire pit and provided wood, which Jay really appreciated, especially compared to the last site. Apparently, different parts of the park had different rules for using fire pits.

Jay managed to get a fire going while Milly set up her things.

Once he finished setting up the fire, Jay began working on his own setup. He retrieved the supplies he had packed for his supper and brought them back over to the fire. Milly was already there, heating up her meal. It seemed she was preparing pasta.

"What are you making for supper?" Jay asked.

"Spaghetti with chicken and alfredo sauce." The words rolled off her tongue like cooking a gourmet meal out in the woods was normal. Jay's silence drew her attention, and when she saw Jay's stunned face, she laughed.

"What?! It's good! What did you bring?" She laughed and finished adding her pasta to the boiling water.

"I bet it's good; it sounds delicious. I'm just shocked you brought such a fancy meal. All I brought was a can of stew."

Jay looked down at the can in his hand and give a mock face of disgust, making Milly laugh harder.

"It's not all that complicated. The pasta is hard and won't spoil, and neither will the can of chicken. I just put the alfredo sauce in a plastic container; it won't spoil after one night." Milly smiled as she shook her head and went back to cooking.

Jay was again struck by how beautiful she was. When he was able to hold her hand, something just clicked for him. Something told him this woman was the woman he had been dreaming of for years. She was easygoing and always smiling, laughing at his terrible jokes and a joy to hang out with.

After supper, they both put their food safely up in the storage tree.

Jay smiled, realizing how special Milly was. He wanted her to feel just as special as he saw she was.

A plan had started to form in his head earlier in the night, so he figured now was a good time to put it into action.

The sun had set, and the fire was lighting the surrounding area. There was a flat space off to the side that was clear of any trees, so Jay pulled out his sleeping bag and spread it out on the ground.

Milly watched him with a curious gaze.

"What are you doing?" Milly asked Jay. "You're braver than I if you are planning on sleeping out in the open without a bug net. I hate the feeling of bugs crawling on me." She shivered at the thought.

"Nope, I'm setting up a place to stargaze."

Milly blinked at Jay a few times and then shook her head in disbelief.

"What?" said Milly.

Jay laughed at her confused expression. It was a little odd to unzip your whole sleeping bag and lay it on the dirt to look at the stars, but Jay didn't have anything to make it more comfortable, so he did what he could.

"Would you like to stargaze with me, Milly?" he asked her.

Still slightly stunned, it all must have suddenly clicked in her mind because a small smile crossed her face and her cheeks turned bright red, which Jay very much liked seeing.

"Ok," she said, coming over to the makeshift blanket area and sitting on the edge. She removed her boots and turned a little, but couldn't seem to put her feet on the sleeping bag.

Jay sat down beside her but looked at her feet. "What's wrong?" he asks.

"Nothing! I just... do you really want me to put my sweaty feet on your sleeping bag? I've been hiking all day."

Her cheeks were pink again, showing she was embarrassed by the truth in her statement.

"I am one hundred percent sure I want your sweaty feet on my sleeping bag. Besides, mine are far worse!" She laughed at Jay's comment and slowly put her feet on the sleeping bag.

Jay rearranged himself and lay on his back to look up at the sky. Milly sat upright with her head tilted back to see the stars.

"Milly." Jay's soft voice was carried to Milly's ears. She turned to look at him, and Jay stretched out his arm, inviting her to lie down with him. She tried to hide the smile on her face and failed, which brought a lot of joy to Jay.

She scooted closer to Jay and lay down on her back, resting her head on his arm. This felt so right to Jay. Milly brought so much peace to his constantly racing mind.

"This is the calmest I have felt in a really long time," Jay said while still looking at the sky.

"Really? Is your life really that busy?" she asked.

Jay had to stop and think about that for a moment.

"I don't think that it's busy, but rather it's loud. Sure, I am always going to and from work, but when I'm at home, even alone, there is still traffic out the window or noise in the hall of my apartment building. I think the city is meant to be loud and busy. I just don't think I want to be part of it anymore," Jay explained, looking down at Milly, who had her head tipped up towards him.

Her chocolate-colored eyes held Jay's gaze, drawing him in like a magnet. He found himself unable to look away, lost in their depth.

"Let me ask you the same. What do you want for your life? Are you happy with where you are?" he asked.

Jay's question hung in the air, waiting for Milly's response. There was a brief pause as Milly wrestled with her thoughts, trying to decide whether to open up to him.

"Honestly?" Milly finally spoke, her voice tentative yet sincere.

"Yes, honestly." Jay's response carried a gentle encouragement, hoping to coax Milly into sharing her thoughts with him. He was genuinely interested in understanding her aspirations, craving insight into her world.

"My dream has always been to have a family and live in my small town. It's not a glamorous dream, but anytime I think of my future, I want it to be one surrounded by kids and someone to love."

Milly's admission was laced with vulnerability, revealing her deepest desires. As she spoke, nerves fluttered within her, but Jay's comforting touch on her cheek soothed her.

Jay's thumb caressed her cheek very gently, a tender gesture of both understanding and support.

"That sounds like a perfect dream," Jay whispered as he slowly leaned down to kiss Milly.

He went slowly enough to give her enough time to move away if she didn't want to kiss, but she didn't move. She leant up and brushed Jay's lips with hers.

The moment was sweet and intimate. Jay was amazed at how his weekend has transformed into something so incredible and special.

He had begun thinking he would be on his own, but instead, he had stumbled upon this marvelous woman.

After their kiss, they held hands and continued gazing up at the stars.

Jay felt certain that this was just the beginning of something amazing. So, when they eventually retired to their own sleeping bags, Jay rested, his mind set on what he wanted to do next.

Chapter 6
New Adventures

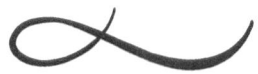

THE FOLLOWING morning came around far too quickly for Milly's liking, as she didn't want the weekend adventure to end. Milly and Jay walked most of the way back, hand in hand when possible. Milly found Jay's presence comforting and warm.

The kiss the night before was etched in Milly's memories and was likely to remain there for the whole of her life.

She couldn't have imagined a more perfect setting for their first kiss.

One of her favorite things to do was to lie under the stars, and though Jay had no idea that was the case, it had fulfilled a dream of hers.

Milly thought Jay was a kind and caring person, as he had asked questions about her family and life, always remembering details she had shared earlier. It felt like a dream, and Milly couldn't shake the fear that it might indeed be just that—a dream.

They made it back to the parking lot close to evening. Milly was surprised to find out they both had parked in the same lot.

Jay walked with her over to her car and helped her put her pack inside. Milly felt herself melting inside at how gentle he was with her, how tenderly he treated her.

"I guess this is where we part," Milly said with a sad smile. They hadn't talked about staying in touch, so as far as Milly knew, this was just a magical weekend to remember although she hoped for more.

Jay stepped a little closer to Milly, taking both her hands in his.

"I've had the best weekend. I knew the hike would be great, but you turned it into something special," Jay said, his voice filled with sincerity. "I know we've just met, but can I call you? Maybe see you again?"

Milly's heart beat a little faster. She was thrilled to hear that Jay had also enjoyed the weekend.

"I would love that. A lot, actually," she replied, her smile widening.

Jay smiled back at her and kissed her, but this time, he wasn't so timid about it; he kissed her, showing her how much he liked her. This time, it showed her that he knew what he wanted - and he wanted her.

After exchanging numbers, they went their separate ways, happy in the knowledge that this was the beginning of something special.

Over the next few months, they talked on the phone every night.

Milly brought happiness to Jay's busy life; she was a living reminder that he could have the quiet life he so desperately wanted. The calls lasted so long as neither of them wanted to end them.

They discussed their days at work, their thoughts on different news stories and about music, celebrities, new camping equipment and much more. They each felt comforted hearing the other's voice.

At the end of each phone call, they said goodnight to each other, several times over before ending the call and realising how long and lonely the next 24 hours would be.

Jay visited her often on the weekends and fell in love with Newhill.

He agreed that the world seemed to pass Newhill by and that the village always seemed incredibly quiet, but as he pointed out to Milly, time there was probably marked by the passing seasons rather than the hands on a clock.

Milly introduced him to her parents, who absolutely adored him. They enjoyed his company and Milly's mom loved to prepare a leisurely lunch for them to enjoy.

Milly's father would often recall the times he and Milly went camping and these included tales of when ants found their way into their breakfast oats and when the double air mattress they used got a puncture and they both had to sleep on the lumpy and incredibly cold ground.

On one occasion, her father disappeared for ages as he searched in his study for the albums of old photographs of the various camping expeditions.

Jay noticed that Milly was smiling in all the aging photographs – including several when it was raining hard.

Milly also visited the city to see Jay, and he took her around to show her all the cool spots, including the best Chinese restaurant in the area.

They would spend hours walking around or jumping on and off buses to see the various sites, but in the evening over their meal, Milly would tell Jay that although she occasionally enjoyed the buzz of city life, the slower pace of the life she led was preferable.

One weekend, Jay decided to introduced Milly to his friend Ben and his family. It was a great weekend where they enjoyed some of the city's finer things that were aimed at children and Jay noticed how well Milly coped with the demands of young children.

On the Monday at work, Ben had expressed how much he and his wife had enjoyed the weekend too and how lovely they though Milly was – they were a great match, Ben had proclaimed!

By fall, Milly missed Jay every time he had to leave. They had fallen in love, and she longed to be with him.

They had plans that weekend; Jay was coming to visit again. After Milly finished work, she hurried home to get things prepared in her apartment ready for Jay.

At five o'clock, the doorbell rang at her small apartment. Milly rushed to the door and swung it open to find the very person she knew would be standing there.

She threw herself at Jay, who caught her easily.

"I missed you!" Milly exclaimed into his neck as she squeezed him tightly.

"I missed you more," Jay replied, returning the tight embrace. It had become a running joke between them; who missed whom more? They obviously hadn't decided who won that one yet.

"You ready to go? I have a surprise for you," Jay exclaimed. Milly was bouncing up and down with excitement. She loved surprises.

Jay drove to the other side of town, down a quiet street. Milly didn't understand why they were there; the area was residential, nothing too special about it.

They pulled up to a smart bungalow at the end of the street. It was a lovely place, Milly thought. Climbing out of the vehicle, Jay came around to Milly's side. He took her hand and walked up to the sidewalk that led up to the front door. Milly was getting nervous; she didn't think they were visiting someone today.

"What do you think of the house?" Jay asked.

"It's lovely, but... what are we doing here?" Milly replied.

"This is my house," he said.

Milly whipped her head around and looked up into Jay's smiling face.

"Are you serious?" Milly's said with excitement. She hoped he wasn't kidding because she desperately wanted him to live closer to her.

"Yeah, I just got the keys today. Of course, I don't have anything in it, but it's mine." He dangled the keys in the air to show Milly.

Milly jumped up and down, hugging Jay.

"I am so happy for you! I can't believe you are finally going to be closer to me! Wait! What are you going to do for a job?" Milly asked, concerned.

"I quit my job a few weeks ago; this was my last week. I got a job at the real estate office here in town. I didn't tell you because I wanted it to be a surprise," he said.

"I am surprised!" said Milly as she smiled up at him.

"Come on, there's more," Jay said as he started pulling her along behind the house.

"How could this get better?" Milly said, seemingly unable to contain her excitement.

Behind the house, a path led directly to the covered bridge that crosses over the small river in town. The bridge was adorned with decorative string lights lining the edges.

Milly had always loved the bridge and thought it was a romantic spot. Once they reached the middle of the bridge, Jay turned to look at Milly.

Milly's heart beat faster with anticipation as they approached the bridge. She couldn't help but wonder what Jay had planned.

While a part of her hoped for a proposal, she didn't want to get her hopes up. Then, Jay dropped to one knee, and tears welled up in Milly's eyes.

"Milly, from the first time I saw you sitting on that camping platform, I knew my world had changed. That weekend hiking with you was one of the best times of my life, and I can't imagine my life without you. You've become an intricate part of it. I want more hiking adventures and trips together, but mostly, I want to wake up one morning with you in my arms as my wife."

The tears flowed down Milly's cheeks as a swell of love filled her heart.

"Milly, will you marry me? Will you be my hiking buddy? Will you start a family with me and grow old together?"

Milly didn't hesitate; she dropped to her knees too and hugged Jay tightly, saying 'yes' over and over again.

Jay slipped the ring onto her finger, sealing their commitment to each other. A chance encounter had transformed their ordinary lives into something truly extraordinary.

Epilogue
10 Years Later

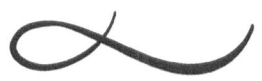

"ANDREW, can you grab the small cooler from the trunk?" Jay asked his oldest son who had been standing quietly watching his father as he worked.

"Sure, Dad!"

Milly and Jay had been happily married for ten years. A year after their wedding, they welcomed their son Andrew into the world.

Three years later, Willa joined the family. She was a vibrant and energetic little girl, always eager to explore her surroundings and meet new people. Now six years old, she was full of smiles and laughter and would often skip along, her pigtails and ribbons dancing in the breeze as she went.

In complete contrast, her older brother, who was nine years old, was more serious and thoughtful. He loved to understand how everything worked from how baby birds learnt to fly to how television pictures were created.

Jay finished setting up the two-person tent for the kids as Milly carefully hung the double hammock they would share between two sturdy trees.

"DAD! Look, I found a frog!" Willa rushed over to Jay, showing him the small slimy frog she found at their campsite.

"Good job, honey. Why don't you put it back where you found it and then wash your hands? I bet Mom would love your help putting the sleeping bags in the tent," Jay suggested as Milly grabbed the kids' sleeping bags.

"Okay!"

Willa rushed off to do just that. Jay started a fire and began preparing supper, Milly came over to sit beside him.

"Need any help?" Milly's sweet smile hadn't changed in all the years they had been together, and it still made Jay happy to see her every day.

"Sure, want to start boiling the water for the pasta?" A staple for their family camping trips was pasta, Alfredo sauce, and canned chicken. Jay often laughed, saying they were eating gourmet food, reminding Milly of their second night at Kisik Grotto.

Time passed quickly, as it usually did, and soon enough, the kids had climbed into their sleeping bags to go to sleep.

Milly and Jay found themselves sitting alone by the campfire, the quietness bringing a sense of peaceful calm to the night.

"I can't believe how far we've come," Milly said wistfully, looking at the flames of the fire. Jay reached for her hand and squeezed it lightly.

"The best thing that ever happened to me was stumbling upon you at that park. I would hate to think how my life wouldn't have changed if I hadn't met you. I probably would still be in the city, unhappy with my corporate job and finding very little peace," Jay admitted.

"And I would probably still be a receptionist and hiking alone at the weekends. I'm happy that's not what my life is, though. I love the kids and I love you too," Milly said warmly, gently squeezing his hand.

The fire crackled as they sat together, watching the flames dance. As the night progressed, the stars emerged, shining down on them, witnessing the love of a family grow and grow.

The End

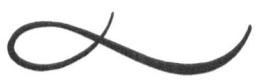

Other Books from Seniorality

To find your next book Seniorality book visit:

www.amazon.com/author/seniorality

Where you will find:

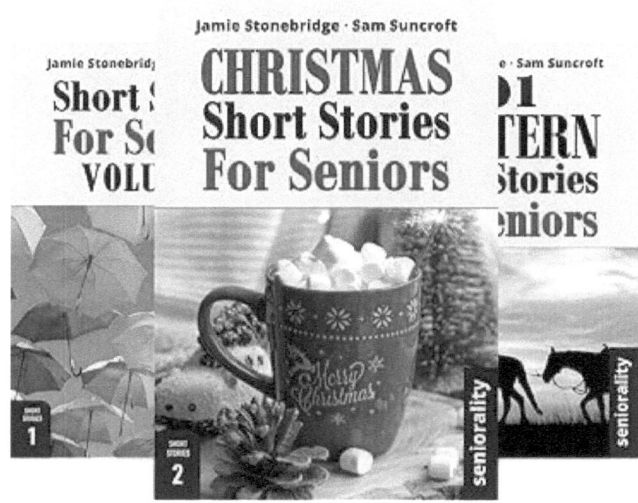

Short Stories

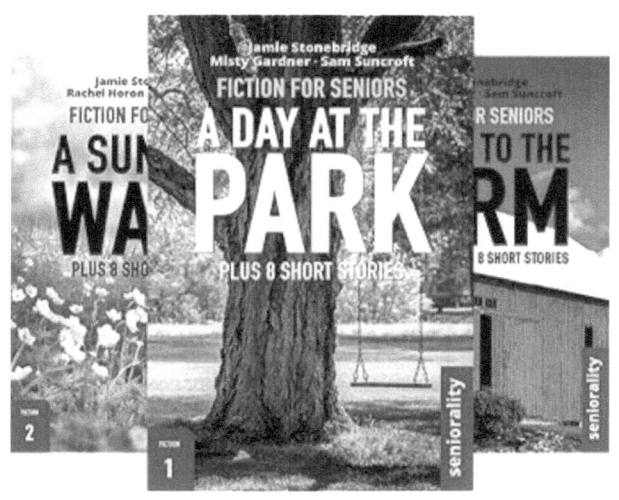

Fiction for Seniors

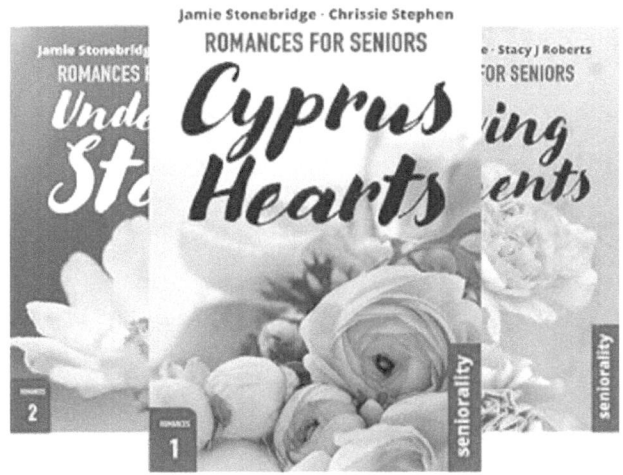

Romances for Seniors

Find these and many more books
by searching on Amazon for 'seniorality'
or visit: **www.amazon.com/author/seniorality**

Thank You

If you enjoyed this book or found it useful, we'd be very grateful if you'd post a short review on Amazon.

Your support really does make a difference and helps other people discover this book.

We personally read all reviews to hear how the books are being used, to collect feedback, and get ideas for future stories.

Thank you and have a wonderful day!

www.ingramcontent.com/pod-product-compliance
Lightning Source LLC
Chambersburg PA
CBHW031924240526
45464CB00022B/809